I KNOW WHAT IT'S LIKE...
AN OVARIAN CANCER STORY

JENNIFER COURT

Ant Press
Large Print
Edition

LARGE PRINT EDITION

Copyright © 2022 by Jennifer Court

Illustrations by Sheila Tolbert

First Edition, 2022

Published by AntPress.org

ISBN Paperback: 978-1-922476-60-9

ISBN Hardback: 978-1-922476-61-6

ISBN Large Print Paperback edition: 978-1-922476-62-3

ISBN Large Print Hardback edition: 978-1-922476-63-0

For my husband John, whose love, patience and understanding throughout my cancer journey has been immeasurable.

And for all Ovarian Cancer patients and survivors...
I know What It's like.

CONTENTS

I KNOW WHAT IT'S LIKE

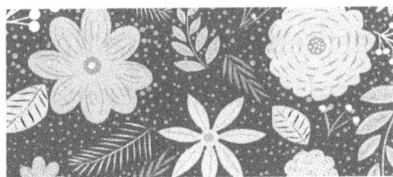

I know what it's like to hear the news
That cancer has entered your life.
Everything turned upside down
New normal filled with strife.

I know what it's like
To play the waiting game...
Are numbers trending up or down,
Or will they stay the same?

I know what it's like to distance yourself
From family and well-meaning friends.
For fear that they will pass down germs
That'll sicken your body, once again.

BUT...

I also know what it's like to hear,
Your numbers are okay.
And treatments seem to do their job
To take the cancer away.

I know what it's like to cling to support
And cherish newfound hope.
And when my fortitude returned,
It helped me climb that slippery slope.

No one has a crystal ball
To see what our future has in store.
But...I know what it's like to think positive
thoughts,
When cancer will be no more!

OVARIAN CANCER — SAY WHAT?

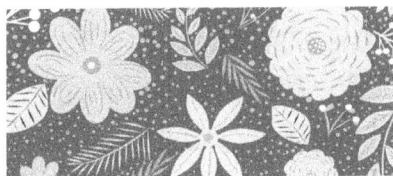

When I was only forty-three
My life began to spin.
Surgery, Cancer and Chemo
Took away my wind.

Our oldest left for college
How could I say goodbye?
My other one in High School
Watched through tears in eyes.

When the chemo was complete
I happily rejoiced.
Thanked God and all my doctors
Who gave this powerful voice.

While traveling through my therapy
I searched both high and low.
For anything "Ovarian"
Just simply wanted to know.

Could not find any words or books
To bring such knowledge to me.
So, I wrote this story
For all who want to seek.

Because of my experience I know what it is
like.
To receive an unexpected lift to get one
through the night.
For all who are downtrodden, please accept
this lift.
Here is my story...
Here is my gift!

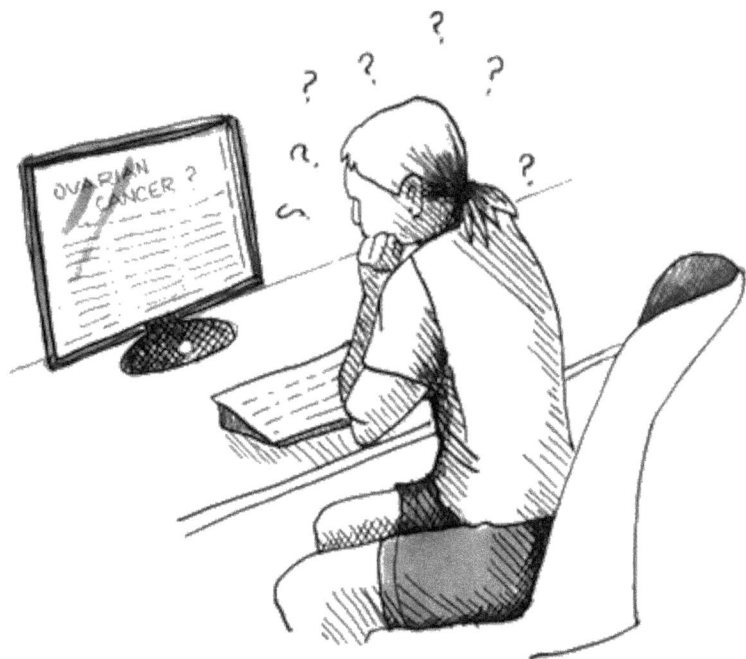

CHAPTER I

~ JULY, 2000 ~

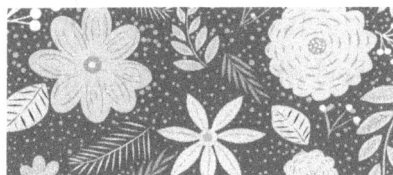

I remember that fateful day in the spring of 2000. I was at a health booth at our local Community Center, going through the motions to get points for my husband's insurance plan. After all, I was forty-three and the picture of good health.

When the lady behind the counter quizzed me about stress in my life, I answered honestly, "The only stress that I can think of is that my older son is going away to college in the Fall. I'm basically a happy go-lucky girl. No need to worry about me."

Wow! That memory sure comes back to haunt me.

One night in July, I wondered why my

stomach kept growing larger. After dinner with friends, I laid down on my back and pointed out my abdominal area, which looked like I was four months pregnant. Every person gains weight in a specific location, but mine is typically not in my stomach. Concerned enough to call my doctor the next day, I was able to get an appointment right away and was told that I had an ovarian cyst.

"Does it need to come out?" I asked nervously.

"Yes, it is the size of a beach ball!" the doctor replied.

First, an ultrasound of my abdomen was needed. At that time, we lived in a small Wisconsin town of three thousand and they were able to fit me in about an hour later. The technician gasped as he performed the procedure. I must have asked what was wrong, so he caught himself and said that my stomach was really full from all the water they had me drink for the ultrasound. Naively I believed him but later learned that was just the beginning.

My husband John and I met with the local surgeon, a few hours later.

"When do I need to have surgery?" I asked.

His reply was, "Yesterday!"

That shocked the daylights out of us, so we agreed to have it two days later at our local hospital. He did not think it was cancer and if it was, it would be a low-grade form. I felt like he was speaking a foreign language but his cool demeanor and great reputation were comfort enough. Small town hospitals do not have the specialists that metropolitan clinics have. In hindsight, we should have asked for a second opinion in the Twin Cities, which was only two hours away.

The day before surgery, I had a pre-op appointment. The nurse asked if I realized that a complete hysterectomy was scheduled. I nodded my head yes. She also said under her breath that the surgeon must be suspecting cancer. It felt like someone kicked me in the stomach but I would worry about that when the results came in.

Our older son had a two-day college orientation scheduled on the same day as my surgery. UW- Madison was four hours away, so I told John if the results were good, the two of them should take off anyway. I wanted to make sure Dan could get into his chosen classes and assured John that there was a myriad of people to take care of me. After surgery, John came in to say that everything looked good, so I groggily told him to take off.

When I woke up later that day, my younger son Tim was sitting in a chair next to my bed. There is truly nothing like family and my heart was overflowing with happiness and pride.

That evening a friend of mine came to check on me. We visited for a while and I asked her to please turn on Survivor, which was in its inaugural season, before she left. I remember falling asleep in mid-sentence and when I awoke a few hours later, my friend was gone but Survivor was on the television. There is not much I remember about that episode, except that Gretchen was voted off. The power of reality TV!

I was in the hospital for about five days and had visitors coming and going. Every summer my husband's bridge group had a golf outing and because I had never played the game, the excuses were mounting on why we would miss it once again. When I

I KNOW WHAT IT'S LIKE...

called a friend to tell her that we would not be there for the fifth year in a row, she asked what my excuse was this time.

"Does major surgery qualify?" I asked.

She was shocked, but five minutes later this friend and her husband showed up in my hospital room. The power of a small town!

A few days after returning home, I received the news that I had ovarian cancer. It was not a big surprise but when you are told to make an appointment with an oncologist, that shakes you to the proverbial core.

We decided that it was time to see a doctor in the Twin Cities, but while waiting for an opening, we met with a local oncologist in a nearby town for the first opinion. It was hot and I swear the air conditioning was broken in the clinic. Because my abdomen was still sore from surgery, I was tired and cranky waiting for the doctor to arrive.

After he came in, I shut my eyes and listened while he talked about the "protocol" for chemotherapy. He mentioned that even though the stage was unknown, he would still treat it with chemotherapy. At that remark, my eyes shot open and I questioned why they did not know what stage it was in. Apparently, someone at a larger hospital mixed up one of my tests with another patient's. The only way to repeat the test was to open me up again. I was livid, and the hospital would not acknowledge that someone had made a mistake.

Seeing as additional surgery was the farthest thing from my mind, we met with a caring gynecologic oncologist the next week at Abbott Northwestern in Minneapolis. She agreed to take me on as her patient and for the first time in two weeks, I felt that everything was under control. The power of a big city!

The following Friday, we left in the wee hours of the morning for the drive to Minneapolis. Our appointment was early because it took about eight hours from the time we saw my doctor until the time we were released. To start things off, my blood was tested to see if the levels were high enough to receive chemotherapy.

After meeting with the doctor, a chemo nurse inserted an IV into the top part of my hand. In my opinion, oncology nurses are one of God's gifts to cancer patients, as they are patient, kind and understanding. I have terrible veins, so one of the nurses wrapped my hand in warm towels to get them to pop out. Next, a bag of Benadryl was inserted into my IV as a precaution for any allergic reaction to the chemotherapy. It also made me sleepy which, as one can imagine, was an added bonus.

After that, the fun really began - just kidding! They hooked up the chemo drugs to my IV and right away I started to feel a little off kilter. Let's just say that the best part of the entire day was the warm towels and food they brought around in a little cart. My favorite treat was animal crackers. To this day, I still eat them but have switched to the delicious chocolate flavor.

Because we had a two-hour ride home, our doctor suggested that we ask one of the nurses to administer another bag of Benadryl to make me sleepy during that stretch. To me, that was a miracle drug. It was hard to believe that this would be my life every three weeks for a total of six treatments.

Everything was happening so quickly. How did I get to this point?

I felt pretty good for a few days but decided to take the anti-nausea drug Compazine to ward off any side effects that were headed my way. That was a huge mistake for me. After taking them for 24 hours, the side effects made me crazy. I have never used illegal drugs but now know what taking "speed" feels like.

John and I ended up in the emergency room, where the doctor told me to stop taking the drugs and said that I would feel better after they left my system. He was right and I actually felt pretty good until my next appointment three weeks later.

Unfortunately for me, I seemed to get most of the side effects from the chemo and it soon looked and felt like my hair would be a thing of the past. I was determined to keep it until we dropped Dan off at Madison two days before my second appointment, as I did not want his last memory of his mom to be sickly and bald. Hey, even I was freaked out looking at myself in the mirror. Before we took Dan to Madison, I discovered a letter that was left lying around his bedroom that he wrote to himself. The only thing that stuck out in my memory was that he talked about my cancer and that he was not ready to lose me. Apparently, I taught him such things as, "To have a good friend, you have to be a good friend." and "When in doubt, go to Disney World!"

On the day that we drove Dan south to Mad town, with my Badger red bandana covering my head, the entire family delivered him to college. It was a bittersweet moment for me but my son was a trooper. Before we left, he gave me a hug, looked at me with his big, uncertain eyes and went off to meet new kids. By that time, my head was itchy and the bandana was turned almost sideways. In other words, I looked a mess on what was probably the hottest day of the summer.

We stopped at a McDonalds halfway home but before we got out of the car, my husband chuckled and said, "I hate to say it but your hair looks awful."

It was pretty funny, and when we arrived home that night, I asked, "Who wants to help me pull the hair out of my head?"

John thought I should pull it out while in the shower but that seemed like too much to clean up. So, under the stars and moon, I quickly tugged on my hair and it easily came out. That was the most liberating feeling as my head finally cooled off. It felt so good that I thought John and Tim were going to have to get used to my baldness. Definitely comfort before beauty!

Before surgery, my sister Jody (who lived in Texas at the time) persuaded me to get a CA125 test. She had just heard about it that morning and learned that it showed the possibility of ovarian cancer. The normal range is thirty-five or below. Mine registered at sixty-five. That is one of the tests that they do before each chemo treatment.

While receiving the second round of chemo, I learned that my CA125 count dropped to five. What a relief, the drugs were working!

The side effects from each round of chemo became more and more prevalent. I was never sick to my stomach but one nurse likened it to feeling like you were run over by a Mack truck. Each second of the day seemed like a minute, each minute like an hour and each hour like a day. Only time (as in days) made me feel a little better. One of the side effects for me was constant constipation. Fortunately, just hearing my friend Sue's voice on the phone, as well as over-the-

I KNOW WHAT IT'S LIKE...

counter drugs, helped alleviate that problem. Before one of my treatments, I came down with a cold and my white blood count was too low to receive chemo. It made me nervous to delay it a week, thinking that it might disrupt the progress. I thought how odd it was that I wanted so badly to be healthy enough to receive chemo, so that more pain and suffering could be inflicted upon my already ravaged body.

Jody came to stay with me for a week in September. During that time a friend stopped by to cut off the little wisps of hair that I was unable to pull out on that August summer night. Jody sighed at the tragedy of the situation. I persuaded her not to worry as it was saving us money to keep the air conditioner off during the hot, Indian summer days. I was a big fan of president movies so we watched them all from Murder at 1600 to Dave to The American President. To this day they are still some of my favorites. Just having Jody around lifted my spirits and I was ready to continue the fight.

In early October, my friend Carol came over from New Hampshire to help out for a week. I felt pretty good because it was the week of my treatment when I felt the strongest and best. She decided that we were going to make my ten batches of Christmas cookies which is always a huge undertaking for me. For all of my friends and family, don't worry if you received them that year, as they were safely stored in the deep freezer!

Carol has endless energy so we also cleaned, cooked and walked until we dropped. Toward the end of the week she accompanied John and me to my third treatment. That proved to be a blessing, as she took my mind off of the pain and worry and gave John a much-needed break from the whole mental process.

Also, by the third treatment, my CA125 level dropped to one. My doctor was thrilled and wondered if I really needed chemotherapy drugs. I cheerfully asked her if we were done but she replied that I had to finish the regimen of six rounds. With such good numbers, it was a small price to pay for a clean bill of health.

Before John and I were married, we decided that Northern Wisconsin or Minnesota would be a great place to raise a family. We received our wish with John working for two wonderful companies in both of those states. When you live in Wisconsin, you almost always become a Green Bay Packer, Milwaukee Brewers and Wisconsin Badgers fan. Our friends Billie and Jerry gave us three tickets to a Monday night Packer/Vikings rivalry football game in early November at Lambeau Field. The weather forecast called for rain which made me crazy worried about going for fear of catching a cold, as I did not want to delay another treatment. John convinced me that this was a chance of a lifetime, so we drove the five hours to Green Bay and watched the Packers win with a miracle shoestring catch by Antonio Freeman in overtime! John, Tim and I happily listened to the post-game show the entire ride home. It was an unforgettable night mixed in amongst the gloom and pain that I will forever cherish.

My son Tim was a junior in high school during this turmoil. He patiently understood what was going on and helped out whenever possible. Except for school, he rarely left our home. Tim and several of his friends took AP History and they spent almost every school night at our house studying. We had a walkout basement with a refrigerator and oven in the laundry room. They entered through the downstairs door and ate pizzas throughout the evening. Their constant chatter helped ease my mind, although I felt a little guilty that pizza was Tim's staple food in his diet.

The girls came upstairs to check on my health which made me feel special. In a weird way, I look back at those days with fond memories.

As the weather got colder, we cranked up our fireplace. Sometimes, it was so warm down in the basement that I could hardly breathe and felt like it was actually my body that was on fire. I learned that at those strange times I was experiencing hot flashes. Nobody explained that when I had the hysterectomy in July, my body went into instant menopause. Although I had heard of menopause and hot flashes, unless you have been through both of them, you cannot possibly understand how women feel. I almost felt like I was dying, because the hot flashes were so peculiar.

During the months of treatments, I was afraid to go out to a public place, for fear of getting sick. Carol and her husband Mark came back to Minnesota for Thanksgiving and wanted to visit for a night. We decided that I should venture out, so we headed over to my favorite "Up North" restaurant called The Five O'clock Club for dinner. One of Carol's friends sent some beautiful scarves for me to borrow for my bald head. Up to that point, I had only been wearing red and blue bandanas or nothing at all. So, it was a treat to have her style one of them into a "funky" turban and away we went. Halfway through supper, I could feel the scarf coming loose and it completely fell apart. Horrified, I held on with both hands and then all four of us laughed at the humorous situation.

One of my favorite memories of this traumatic experience took place around the same time. Dan asked if he could bring a friend home from his dorm for Thanksgiving. It was fine with me but I told him there would not be much homemade food around, like usual. Ben is from Oregon and he quickly became a member of our family and is like a third son to me. Dan swears that they are twins that were separated at birth.

Every Thanksgiving, no matter where

everyone is located, we always have a football pool for the two holiday games. The only participants are Dan, Tim, John and Ben. After drawing names for the order of selection, they pick their teams. For the last several years we have needed a conference call, as the boys have all gone their separate ways. One year, Dan was on his honeymoon in Thailand but managed to find time for that all-important call. There is now a traveling bobblehead turkey trophy for the victor. Dan's wife Sarah was happy to give it up to the next winner (Tim) as I am pretty sure that it did not match their home decor!

My last treatment was in December. The days that I felt good between them were almost non-existent. The side effects on my body were cumulative but I was buoyed by the fact that the misery would soon end. We were thankful for my doctor and the nurses who patiently took good care of me.

Because my husband works for a turkey company, we brought a deli-tray for all to share. It is funny how safe I felt as long as the chemicals were going into my body and were killing off any cancer cells. Once the treatments stopped, I started to feel vulnerable that the cancer was not completely gone and the cells would start multiplying again.

After a follow-up CT scan, a spot was discovered on my liver. A month later, the scan was repeated. Although the spot was still there it was determined to be benign. Yahoo, I was officially cleared! It was time to thank my family and friends.

I decided to host a "Survivor" party to let everyone know how much their help was appreciated during this trying period of my life. First, I needed to compile a list of people to invite. When looking back, I was overwhelmed by the amount of family, friends and acquaintances who came to my aid.

One friend brought me chicken dumpling soup every three weeks to coincide with my treatments. It was one of the few healthy foods that tasted good to me.

Another friend and her mom did the same thing with homemade cinnamon rolls. A multitude of people from our town knew that my first love was chocolate so there was never a shortage of sweets around. It was no surprise that I gained six pounds from one treatment to the next. I complained to the nurse on that one saying, "Who gains six pounds in three weeks?"

All she did was smile and assured me that was a good thing.

One day, a Sunday school class from our church showed up to rake leaves. Also, a friend of mine called every week to see what my family needed from Wal-Mart. As it was getting close to Christmas, I gave her a list of DVDs that my boys asked for. I never paid attention to their "ratings" so when they opened them on Christmas day, in front of my in-laws no less, I was horrified to notice that some of them were rated R. Oh well, what were the chances that the boys would watch them while Grandma and Grandpa were still visiting? Besides, Grandma never stayed awake during a movie anyway. You can imagine my beet-red face when I kept looking over to John's mom during one movie and noticed that she never slept a wink!

The theme for my "Survivor" party was from the reality show that gave me so much to look forward to one night a week during treatments. Dan put together a CD with the shows' music as well as Beach Boys and other summer songs. I ordered decorations, paper goods and really cool-looking key chains from Oriental Trading Company. The key chains were used as thank you gifts for all of my guests and there were other door prizes as well.

At the appointed hour, forty "angels" arrived to help celebrate my good health. I only wished that my family and friends from out of state could have been there as they had done so much for me, especially my wonderful mom and two sisters, Robin and Jody who live in Arizona. By the time everyone left, my heart was overflowing with the realization of how many lives I had touched over the years. That warm, fuzzy feeling will stay with me forever.

CHAPTER 2
~ SUMMER 2003 ~

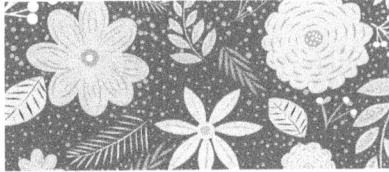

With each three-month checkup, I eagerly awaited the results of the CA125 test. The number continued to stay low, so it seemed that I had beaten Ovarian Cancer. Weight Watchers helped me lose the thirteen pounds I gained and to relearn how to eat healthy foods, at least most of the time. Chocolate snacks continued to be my food of choice for the weekends!

At the time of my cancer treatments, the company that John worked for was in the process of being sold to a larger one located in Minnesota. Because John was an accountant, he was involved in this process. Although he could not fill me in on the specifics, we discussed the possibility and ramifications if the deal "came down". It made the two-hour rides pass quickly and we wondered what else could possibly happen during this unsettled period in our lives.

Well, it did happen and that is why we presently live in Minnesota. John was given a great job with the combination of the two turkey companies but he lived between two states for a year. It worked out well as Tim was able to finish his senior year, so we did not have to move him away from his wonderful group of friends.

One January day, while John was in Minnesota, I read an article in the U.S.A. Today newspaper. It was about ovarian cancer patients who have the BRCA gene mutation and their chances of getting breast cancer, which was over 80%. One of the groups of people that have this particular gene mutation is those of Ashkenazi Jewish descent, affecting Eastern European Jews. Yikes! My parents' families descended from Germany, Russia and Spain. John came home from Minnesota that night and I quickly announced my need for a double mastectomy. His comments were something like, "Back the train up, what are you talking about?"

After showing him the article, he agreed that we should bring it with us to my upcoming doctor visit. When she entered the exam room, we quickly showed her the article and without hesitation she asked if I was Jewish.

"Yes," I replied and then we were told to speak with a genetic counselor and if I tested positive for the gene, she advised me to get the surgery.

With the sale of the company, our insurance changed and we were forced to switch doctors. It was difficult to say good-bye to my oncologist at Abbott Northwestern but felt that Mayo Clinic was a great alternative. So, we began our foray into the incredibly complex clinic in Rochester, Minnesota with an appointment to see a genetic counselor.

A few weeks later, we sat in her office and discussed gene mutations. Because of the young age of my ovarian cancer diagnosis, she explained that there was a good chance the test result would be positive for the BRCA gene mutation. She also asked if I had any sisters or cousins with ovarian or breast cancer. That question brought me back to one of my yearly checkups in Wisconsin. When my physician asked if there were any changes to my family history, I mentioned that a first cousin died from ovarian cancer and another survived breast cancer. He explained that those relationships were not close enough to warrant any concern. In all fairness to that doctor, it never entered my mind that gene mutations were running rampant in my family and that subject was just now making front-page news.

It took all of four minutes for me to tell the genetic counselor that I believed that my test would be positive and that I was prepared to have a double mastectomy. She seemed surprised at my tenacity for this surgery but I never wanted to go through chemo again, so that was that!

Also, my first cousin Bette did indeed have the BRCA I gene mutation, as did my cousin who died from ovarian cancer. If you believe that only females can pass this along, my father, aunt and uncle all passed it down to one child within their family nucleus. And the cycle continues, as I have passed it down to both of my sons. Knowledge is power but also very scary.

Upon hearing that I had the gene mutation, I kept my word and scheduled the double mastectomy for August, between student council camp (where I was a counselor for a week each year) and our trip to take Tim down to UW Madison, where he would be following in his brother's footsteps. That gave me two weeks to recover, plenty of time to recuperate before the empty nesters' trip.

John was a little worried that I elected to have the TRAM flap reconstruction surgery at the same time as the removal. The whole process was expected to take ten to twelve hours with the reconstruction taking the bulk of the time. The abdominal muscles and fat were to be tunneled up to the breast area, where the plastic surgeon would mold them into new breasts. I really liked the idea that he would use my own tissue.

The day before surgery at Mayo Clinic, I met with the plastic surgeon. He marked up my breasts so much that they looked like cattle going to slaughter. It was embarrassing when we went out to dinner that night, as my skimpy summer shirt did not cover some of the marker. It was beginning to look like my body was no longer my own.

The next morning came all too quickly. John and I were passed from nurse to nurse and it seemed that this show would never get on the road. Every nurse asked my date of birth, age, etc. I remember getting a little short with some of them and pointed to my wrist band. John laughed and said this was all necessary. He was right of course, but I was nervous and frustrated.

After a twelve-hour surgery and recovery, I was taken to my room at Methodist Hospital. The only thing I remember from the week was that the tornado siren went off one night which made me feel very frightened. I was pretty sure that my room was not in the hospital basement; which is the only place in the house that I ever feel safe in that situation. Also, my plastic surgeon got a big kick out of John using my empty hospital room during surgery to spread his papers on the floor. It did not surprise me that he squeezed in a days' work while I was on the operating table, as the transition from the sale of the company was taking up much of his time.

When we finally arrived home, John had

to turn around and head back to Minnesota. Fortunately, I knew a few nurses who helped empty the drains coming out of my new breasts. This surgery was so much more painful than the first one and it was clear that I would not be able to accompany Tim to his move-in day at Madison. That is one of the biggest regrets in my life: I wish I would have scheduled the surgery earlier in the summer. When I told this to my plastic surgeon, he replied that I just had four major surgeries and my body would take a much longer time to heal. It did not make me feel any better.

After a few months, I was back on the operating table getting my nipples formed from the skin transferred up during the original surgery. My doctor said it would be a piece of cake but I have since learned there is never a "piece of cake" surgery. Being awake and hearing him call for a scalpel and other such instruments was almost as terrifying as being put under. Several weeks later, I noticed that the healing nipples had scabbed over and fallen off. My doctor was extremely disappointed when that happened because it was a first for him. We tried to console him by saying it was all right as they were not important anyway. He told me to come back in three months to which I replied, "I am good."

He then said, "Come back in six months."

We then bantered back and forth with me telling him, "This is bothering you more than it is me."

We then realized that a plastic surgeon is like an artist and that he probably felt like he failed to complete his piece of work. I am very satisfied with the results. In fact, the only time I wear a bra is usually to exercise or work out.

There were advantages and disadvantages from the reconstruction surgery. Because muscle and fat were used from my abdomen, my stomach stays pretty flat, which is every postmenopausal woman's dream. Before you all rush out for the surgery, remember that all good junk food has to land somewhere and I now have "love handles" where they had never been.

The biggest disadvantage is that to keep me from getting a hernia, a mesh was put in the abdominal area. To this day, when it gets irritated from over-exercising, lifting, standing in one place too long or sitting in hard, straight back chairs, my stomach tries to push out of the mesh and becomes very uncomfortable.

This will follow me forever but again, is a small price to pay for the security that I have done everything possible to keep the cancer away. It took a long time for me to walk straight up and down and without pain.

Billie saw me out and about one day and thought I was a little old lady walking so hunched over. We had a good laugh over that one. When I decided to do the ten-hour long Tram flap surgery, John questioned this decision. My reasoning was that at forty-five, I felt like I was given a new lease on life and wanted to wake up each day in literally my own skin.

Would I do it again? You betcha, as they say up North! After showing them off to numerous friends, they are always amazed at the outcome. I hardly notice the difference anymore and am very thankful. Life was good, until...

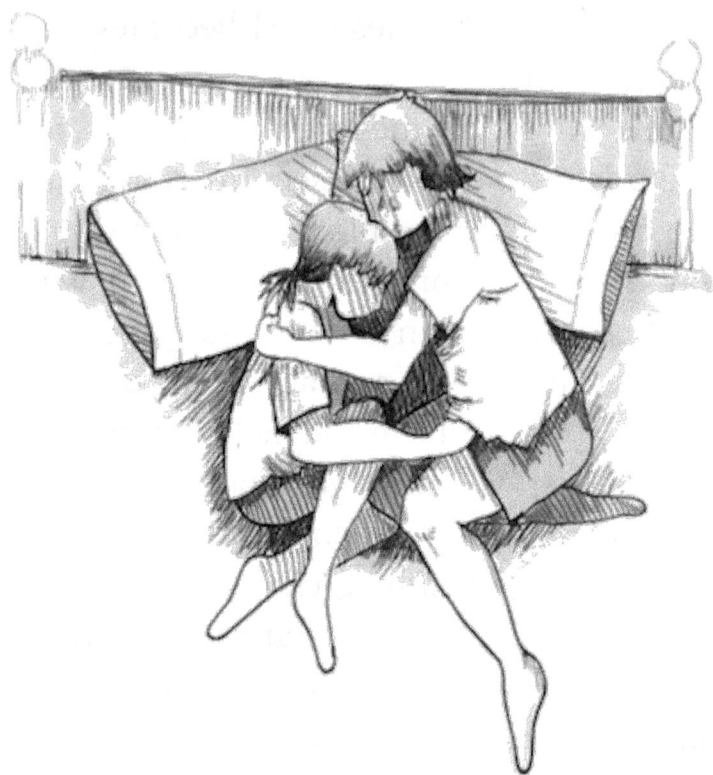

IT'S BACK

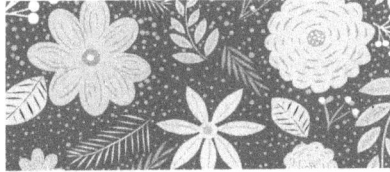

After four plus years of pacified remission
The ugly cancer had returned and forced me
from commission.
Chemo was relentless, made me pitifully sick
Time crawled ever so slowly, the clock barely
ticked.

My blood counts dropped to oblivion
Delayed treatments were the norm.
I always felt incredibly hopeless,
Despondent and forlorn.

John and I had recently moved
To our splendid lake-filled state.
When blinded by this demon again

I questioned my strength to remain.

The turning point for me, was when I said to
John in bed
Told him I was finished and heard him cry
instead.
I turned to him and whispered, "You know
that I will do,
anything to make me whole. It's all because
of you."

So, if the demon comes for you
A knockin' at your door.
Look it squarely in the eye
Then give it hell from your deepest core!

CHAPTER 3

~ 2005 ~

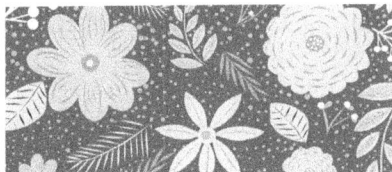

We had been living in Minnesota almost two years when it was time for my four-and-a-half-year check-up at Mayo Clinic in January of 2005. My doctor walked into the room and started asking me several, what I considered strange questions. How do you feel? Can you eat a whole sandwich? Do you get full easily?

I felt great but was frightened nonetheless. She then informed me that my CA125 number went up to fifty-five. My doctor did not seem too concerned and decided to repeat the CA125 test in a month or two and to schedule a CT scan if the levels were still high.

Because the worry gene was passed

down to me from my grandmother, I could not sleep or eat for several days. While talking to Carol about my predicament, she suggested I ask to have a CT scan test right away as it was bothering me so much.

My doctor set up an appointment, so we drove the three plus hours to Rochester, came home and waited for the results. When she called to tell me about three spots on my liver and diaphragm, I was in disbelief. Remembering that there was always a spot on my liver from previous scans, I held out hope that it was simply a routine showing. My husband and I were scheduled to attend a work conference in Long Beach, California the next week until Wednesday, so we made an appointment for the following Thursday. We literally landed at the airport in Minneapolis and drove straight to Rochester.

After a restless night, we met with my doctor. She showed us the CT scan results and I was completely devastated. We then met with a compassionate gynecological surgeon who helped us make the arrangements.

"When do you want surgery?" she asked.

"Tomorrow!" I replied.

She was free but needed a liver specialist

to assist. As she scrolled through the names of those particular doctors, I overheard her mention a familiar sounding one.

"Wasn't that the doctor who performed my breast surgery?" I asked out loud to John.

He thought so too, and my doctor confirmed it. He was also available and agreed to do it the next day. My surgeon kept asking me if I needed anything and my reply was always the same, "Surgery tomorrow!" I think she got a kick out of my persistence to have it "yesterday" but I just felt the need to get the cancer out of my body as soon as possible.

That same night was the longest and toughest of my life. The motel room was dreary and foreboding. John could not bring himself to tell his parents so I was given that job. I also called Jody, who had moved to Arizona and was still at work because of the west coast time difference. We talked for a few minutes and an hour later she called back in tears.

"How did this happen?" she questioned.

I could not give her any answers.

Early the next morning, I was unbelievably back on the operating table. It seemed like I was on the every-other-year-plan for major surgeries and wondered if and when the cycle would stop. Once again, we trusted these surgeons and felt like we were in good hands.

When I awoke, John gave me the thumbs up sign. He said that the tumors were barely attached to the organs and slid right off. My surgeon did have to cut through the mesh (from the reconstruction surgery) so there was a much bigger scar. She also carefully turned over the surrounding organs to check for cancer. I felt good about her diligence.

We decided to have a port implanted above my right breast, which could be used for future chemotherapy. So, a few days after surgery I was back on the table for another one. Fortunately, I was still drugged up from the main surgery and have no recollection of the port implementation.

If you have ever had the misfortune of being cut open, you know that the nurses get you out of bed as soon as possible. A few days later, while I was walking around the corridor, my doctor showed up with one of her students. We called them "docklings". When she asked him to check my scar, he started to look under my gown. She immediately scolded him saying, "Not here! In her room!" Although I had long felt that my body was no longer my own, I was still gratified that my doctor was trying to preserve my dignity. It made me feel good that she cared.

Dan and Tim came to visit from Madison, Wisconsin for the weekend while I was in the hospital. When the nurses came into my room and saw them sleeping on what amounted to fancy folding chairs, they laughed. Only college students can sleep like that!

Whenever I got out of bed to walk, it seemed that my flimsy robe and gown would pop open. Although it was the farthest thing on my mind to cover up immediately, I thought that our kids have definitely seen more of their mother than any children should ever see! At night, they stayed in the motel room with John, and I missed them desperately when they left. I was elated to hear that Jody wanted to come up to Minnesota to help and Carol would fly over the following week.

After I was released from Methodist Hospital, we swung by the Minneapolis airport to collect Jody. She spent the time taking care of me while John was at work and while he slept at night. She cooked, massaged my feet and stayed up with me when I had an adverse reaction to a medication and almost lost my cookies. She also cajoled me into walking around our downstairs family room. It was February, so our walks outside were limited. I cried the day a friend drove her back to the airport.

Fortunately, Carol followed right behind. She picked up where Jody left off, cooking, cleaning, and sitting me on a chair in our freezing garage wrapped in blankets while she cleaned and defrosted our deep freezer. My job was to tell her what to keep and what to throw away. Seems like a crazy thing to do after surgery, but it worked for us. We also walked and giggled the week away. It helped having her with me to ease the gravity of the situation.

One night when we were laughing, John came downstairs to find out what was so funny. I told him that we were planning my funeral with all the trimmings. To get into the service, my guests would have to wear bright clothing. Otherwise, they would not be allowed in the building. Everyone would receive a goodie bag complete with Spaghettios, Hot Tamales and lots of chocolate. There would be tons of fun beach music and decorations to match. John's reply was that we truly were "sick!" It was the kind of thing that kept my spirits up. Humor was never as important as it was during that stressful time.

A good friend of mine moved to Austin, Minnesota six months before my cancer returned. When I mentioned how scared I was to stay in Rochester, she suggested that we stay with her the night before my appointments. What a blessing! Austin is a short forty-five minute drive from Mayo, so in a strange sort of way I actually looked forward to those times. The distraction of three teens and a seven-year-old running around was just what I needed to feel a part of the normal world. LeeAnn would also show up during my chemo treatments and blood transfusions, which was tremendous food for the soul for both John and me.

It was decided that I would receive the same combination of chemo drugs that were used the first go around. I thought that was strange because that regimen did not kill all the cancer cells the first time.

At Abbott Northwestern, the chemo room was one big space with multiple chairs set up for patients. It was similar to a hair salon with IVs instead of hair dryers lying around. Mayo had a similar set up but there were many private rooms available as well. My first treatment was in a private room. I felt claustrophobic and missed the faces of those who were in the same boat as me. One sympathetic nurse told me that I was way too young for this to happen again. Although she meant well, it did not make me feel any better.

My subsequent treatments were in the large rooms and I felt more comfortable from that standpoint. Because it is a three-hour drive from Mayo to our hometown, John asked if they would put another bag of Benadryl in the IV before we went home. They agreed but I got the notion that was not a normal request. During one of my treatments, I became extremely tired and woozy (not in a bad way) before the chemo drugs were even started. We figured out that the nurse thought the two bags of Benadryl were to be given back to back. When my doctor came in asking me a few questions, I explained that it was difficult to focus and concentrate on what she wanted. She left in a huff and said that she would be back later. I am not sure she ever did return!

We never felt comfortable with this doctor from Mayo. She had an assistant who saw me before the treatments so it seemed like being her patient was not a priority. I have a quirky sense of humor that did not mesh with her serious nature. My CA125 number skyrocketed to two hundred twenty-five after the surgery and I was never given a reason why. After three treatments, the number barely went down to the 160's and it seemed to me my life was almost over. My body could no longer tolerate the chemo drugs and I had to be given several units of blood. The serious side effects left off from my previous regimen and I was always nauseous and frightened.

In May, Dan was to graduate with his Master's degree at Madison. After a particularly difficult doctor appointment, John thought we should attend the graduation ceremony that upcoming weekend. He also suggested we head back to Austin from Rochester to see if LeeAnn would help me pick out a wig, thinking that would make me feel more anonymous in a crowd.

I agreed, so around 5:00 LeeAnn, her daughter and I drove to the only open salon in Austin that had any available to purchase. There were two choices. Time was of the essence so I quickly picked out what we called the "Carol Brady" wig. It was not my hair color or style but it was acceptable and we all had a good laugh over the selection.

John went back to work (up north) while I stayed with my friend for two days. Being alone at night made me nervous as I had not been without John since this nightmare began, which might have explained why I had the weirdest dream each night. I groggily woke up to the feeling that the gap between the bedroom curtains was closing. And if it closed completely, I would be dead. Obviously, it was just a dream, but it will never be forgotten.

Two days later, John drove to Austin and we then made our way to Madison. I wore the wig all weekend and it is presently in a Rubbermaid tub somewhere in my closet.

Later, I ordered one from a salon in my area that matched my hair color and style. It was heavily used and even the singed bangs from the campfires could not dampen my spirits while participating in "normal activities".

One stressful night, while lying in bed, I told John that I did not think I could go through this process anymore. Upon hearing him softly cry, I leaned over and said, "You know that I will do everything I possibly can."

"I know you will," he replied.

It was absolutely the lowest point of my life.

We decided to try a different type of chemo that might be easier on my body. The pamphlet that my doctor gave us to read, that incidentally she wrote, gave a warning that the CA125 number might go up after the first treatment. This chemo was given over a two-hour time period and had very few side effects on me. Food still had a metallic taste but there was little nausea and my hair even started to grow back. The CA125 number did indeed go up a little so my doctor was concerned.

After we pointed out the pamphlet warning, I continued with two more sessions. At one August appointment I asked my doctor if we could go on trips in September, October and November. According to her, it would not be a problem, as she would work the treatments around our schedule. When I mentioned how great that would be because I thought I would be dead by then, she said that she would give me two years.

Most of my friends thought that was a heartless answer, when told the story. But it was exactly what I wanted to hear, from the very beginning of this second process, the truth. In addition, two years seemed like a lifetime to me!

Sometime in the summer, John and I were getting more disillusioned with our doctor. I left one appointment in tears after she gave us information about two trial studies that we should think about participating in.

"Am I that bad?" I asked.

Her answer was vague, something about participating in them for other reasons. My husband discovered that his insurance allowed for a second opinion and that our original doctor from Abbott Northwestern was once again on the list of physicians that we could see. With a copy of our latest CT scan in tow, we made our way to the Twin Cities. She looked at the scan and commented that with a "clean" one (meaning no tumors) she would not recommend the studies. There are only so many types of chemo available for ovarian cancer patients and she thought I should wait until they were absolutely needed.

"So, there is hope!" I replied.

She somehow did not commit to that but my spirits were lifted and I felt much better.

After that appointment, John suggested that I call my latest surgeon from Mayo, who we trusted and asked if she knew of any other gynecological oncologists available at the clinic. She asked what I was looking for and I remember my reply as if it was yesterday.

"Someone who will fight for me."

She had the perfect person in mind and I felt like my life had changed forever. My new doctor at the Mayo clinic would become my new best friend.

CHAPTER 4
~ SUMMER 2012 ~

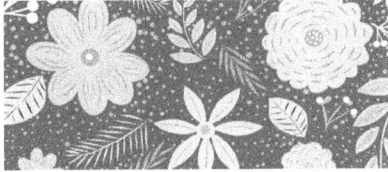

From the moment we met this doctor to the present day, I have felt as though she was heaven-sent. I told her why we switched doctors and her reply was that she had kept a patient alive for twelve years. That was all I needed to know.

We got right to work, any test she wanted me to go through, I happily agreed. Some were not pleasant, but it was worth the time and effort to see if there was any sign the cancer was still there. She decided to put me on tamoxifen, as it is a drug that is sometimes used for breast cancer patients. Because breast and ovarian cancer are related to BRCA gene mutations, we could definitely see the connection. Besides keeping a recurrence away, it is also good for bones which has that extra added benefit.

Although the CT scans continued to be "clean" the all-important CA125 number barely budged. One day, seemingly out of nowhere, the number dropped significantly into the safe zone. We have come up with an unofficial reason which I call the "mesh theory".

Remember that last surgery I had in February, where they cut the mesh in my abdomen? Could all that disruption inside cause the mesh to be irritated and the number to skyrocket? Did the irritation finally settle down after all of those months, causing the number to fall? All valid questions, no particular answer.

Even though we had been in Minnesota for two short years, I had many friends help with my recovery from surgery and during my chemo treatments. My friend Kris drove fifteen miles from a nearby town just to bring me two cans of Spaghettios, my number one comfort food. Another friend brought over a lasagna dinner every three weeks. Others brought salads, helped me clean and toted me to the lab for blood tests.

Our couple friends Sheila & Mike and Annie & Dave kept my spirits up on several Saturday nights. We watched college basketball on our downstairs sectional while drinking wine. I did not feel the best nor did I drink wine but it always felt like such a normal activity, and helped pass the time.

By August, I was ready to thank my new helpful friends. My sister happened to come up for another visit so we planned a luncheon at a local castle for all of my new angels. About fifteen of us ate, laughed and told stories for two hours. When the bill came, my friends wanted to pay their fair shares. I insisted that this was John's treat so the playful arguing ceased.

Unbeknownst to me, Jody confided in Kris that she had been worried about me being in a new town to fend for myself, since we had only lived here a few years. After the luncheon, she felt better about my situation. It was hard to believe how much I had touched those friends' lives in such a short period of time.

Even though my prognosis was not good,

I was still grateful and wanted to celebrate their kindness toward John and myself. I came home with the same fuzzy, warm feeling and realized that there is goodness everywhere.

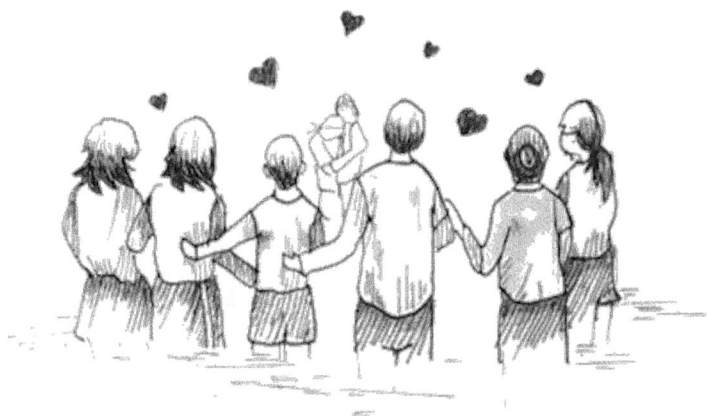

FROM COPE...TO HOPE

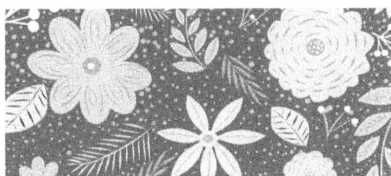

Many people asked, "How did you ever cope?"
Prayers to God I answered, gave me heavenly hope.
Family and friends were present, they helped to rescue me
From nasty side effects of this wretched cruel disease.

Movies, books and TV shows seemed to help the most
Drew my bleak attention from this utterly frightful host.
When Pope John Paul the second, lost his mortal life

I reveled in the moment, when black smoke
turned to white.

Circled myself with positive souls who made
me feel alive
Expressed thanks to these angels, every
single time.
Ones who help unconditionally, are saviors it
is true.
I realized such value when their love came
shining through.

The precious help that saved me, came from
the voice of John
He lifted up my spirits, especially when so
down.
Who saw me at my worst, each and
every day
But said "You are so beautiful" in a very
touching way.

If you are despondent and consumed with
nagging fear
Reach out to your wingman, amongst your
helpful peers.
Lean right in and show her your anguish and
distress

I KNOW WHAT IT'S LIKE...

You will feel much better and finally get some rest!

CHAPTER 5
~ SUMMER 2012 ~

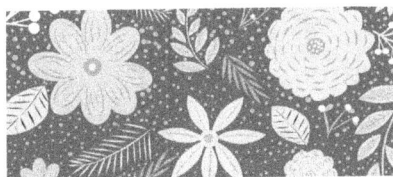

Because my CA125 number seems stable, my doctor visits per year have decreased from every three months to every five. The week before each appointment I find myself imagining that little twinges, aches and pains mean that the cancer is back. That feeling will probably never go away.

So, this section of the story is dedicated to my coping techniques since that fateful day in 2000. Also, included are some goals that I set for myself for the future and changes in appreciation for family and friends.

The biggest way for me to cope with the never ending, rotten feeling days during my treatments was to watch T.V. In 2000, I discovered The Tour de France with Lance Armstrong. Each stage of the bicycle race was filled with anticipation as I watched him grind and race through the mountains and flats.

The Summer Olympics also took place that year. Although I don't remember much about the different sports or athletes, it was a great distraction for two and a half weeks. During my chemo treatments in the year 2005, Pope Jean Paul II passed away and I watched almost every minute of the process to select his successor. I was probably the only one who was happy to see it drag on so long.

Live with Regis and Kelly was a show I looked forward to during the day. They both made me laugh but I particularly loved Kelly's sense of humor on motherhood and just being a woman. The fact that she is a huge ovarian cancer supporter wins big brownie points with me. You go girl!

The year LeeAnn's daughter sold magazines for a school fund-raiser, I jumped at the chance to help out and ordered a three-month subscription to People Magazine. Before cancer, I used to buy an issue to get me through an airplane flight since I am a white-knuckle flier. One day while Dan was visiting, I commented to him and John that my subscription was running out and wondered if renewing it for a year would be a good idea. It was hilarious how they both answered in loud unison, "YES"! It must have kept me from moaning and groaning for a few hours and was well worth the price.

When first diagnosed with ovarian cancer in 2000, one goal I set for myself was to see my son Tim graduate from high school. When the cancer returned in 2005, I had no particular long-range goals. Just keeping my head above water was all I could focus on. Dan moved to the Minneapolis area to start a full-time job at an accounting firm. It was great comfort having him just two short hours away.

That same summer Tim came home for six weeks to help out and to keep my spirits up. He also volunteered at our local newspaper to resuscitate the sports section as sports journalism was his chosen vocation. The two ladies who worked there were happy to have him as they had just discussed how neither of them knew much about that topic. We had a running cribbage game going on which was pretty much one-sided. I am sure you can guess who was the big winner. We also swam together daily.

At the same time, Tim had begun dating Caitlin, a wonderful girl he met at Madison. John and I decided to take him down there for a weekend during this summer stretch. At dinner one night I asked Caitlin if she was a sports fan. Her reply was "not really" and I thought that this relationship will never last. It did last as Caitlin and Tim have been married over three years. She is also a very good athlete participating in triathlons and plays soccer every week.

My next goal was to attend Dan's wedding. But that would require him meeting that special person before the dream could become a reality. The first time I met Sarah I thought that she was wearing a much nicer and trendier outfit than I could ever put together, complete with pointy shoes. Since it seemed Dan did not care about his attire that much, I again thought this relationship would probably go nowhere. And once again, I was wrong. Dan and Sarah have been married over two years and my own personal wardrobe has improved greatly.

A few months after their wedding, John and I prepared for my next five- month check-up. Once I reached that long-term goal, I was more nervous than usual to get the results of my CA125 blood test. Were my sons' marriages the reason that the good Lord was keeping me around? Now that my all-important goals were met, would the cancer appear yet again? To me, these were all valid spiritual questions and I realized more than ever that there was a reason that I continued to live.

Although I was raised in the Jewish faith, John was raised a Methodist. We attended the local Methodist church in Wisconsin because I wanted our boys to grow up believing in God. Our town of three thousand had a multitude of churches but no temples, so we had them baptized and confirmed into the Christian faith. We celebrated both religions' holidays giving them a chance to understand each one. Their friends were jealous during the Christmas and Chanukah seasons as they received presents during most of December. While they were in elementary school, I went into their classrooms to put on Chanukah parties and Passover Seders.

After the second cancer diagnosis, I felt that John would need a church "family" to help him should my health deteriorate. It took a few years before John was ready but we now attend a local Lutheran church. We enjoy the services and being in a house of worship gives me a much-needed sense of inner peace.

In June of 2010 we asked my developmentally disabled brother, Scott, to move to Minnesota from Arizona. Although my sisters and mother lived down there, it was time for a change and we thought our small town would be the perfect place. The downstairs of a house was for rent across the street from us which turned out to be a warm and inviting bachelor pad for my brother.

What can I say about Scottie? His disability is borderline and he is a wonderful, endearing man. Scott drove up to Minnesota in three and a half days by himself. He had been fiercely independent for the past twenty years but it was clear that he needed help and guidance. Although, I am not sure he would agree with that statement!

We love having him so close. He comes over for dinner on Sunday and has lunch with me at least once a week. I introduced him to the local Y.M.C.A and he uses it frequently, often bumming a ride with me. He also delivers pizza about three days a week. Our friends have been wonderful, including him in several social functions and holiday dinners. We have our frustrating moments and days but for the most part things work out and we are super glad to have him "back in our lives." When I mentioned that to him one day he looked at me without batting an eye and said, "I never left!" That is Scott in a nutshell and an entirely different story.

I will always appreciate the wonderful friends that keep entering my life. About four years ago Deb and Herb moved into our townhouse complex and they have been taking care of me ever since, mostly mentally! Maria is my Y.M.C.A. friend and walking partner who with her compassion toward her own developmentally disabled sister in law convinced me that it was a good decision to have Scott move up to Minnesota. We have spent many hours solving not only my problems but the world's, too.

I am reminded of the lyrics to a Girl Scout song "Make new friends but keep the old, one is silver and the other gold." How true. Dan and Tim were an incredible support system. They called every Sunday night from college and continue the tradition today. I recently found engaging emails that were sent during my latest surgery detailing their day to day lives in Madison. I was so concerned about my health at the time that I did not realize how terrifying it must have been for them.

There is not enough time or space to thank everyone. But the one person who I am most grateful for is my dear husband John. Because of the timing of my health problems, he has never been able to experience his own "mid-life crisis" and has stuck by me through thick and thin. I would not be here today without him!

It has been seven plus years since my recurrence was diagnosed. My CA125 number hovers between ten and twenty. I have no idea why it has not come back but I never want to be blind-sided again. Therefore, I prepare myself mentally for recurrent news every five months. That is when my CA125 number is checked at my doctor visit.

My number one philosophy in life is "That there is always someone better off than you and always someone worse off, in every way, shape and form." I feel great and run or walk about eight miles a day. I follow a pretty strict diet during the week but anything goes on the weekend or vacations; remember that I love my chocolate!

A few friends have asked me to speak to other ovarian cancer patients. I am happy to share my story as I realize that I have been given a tremendous gift. Life is unpredictable and I, like other survivors, thrive on hope. Hope that there will someday be a cure and that it will be soon enough to rid all cancer patients of the albatross that is strangling us out of our hopes and dreams.

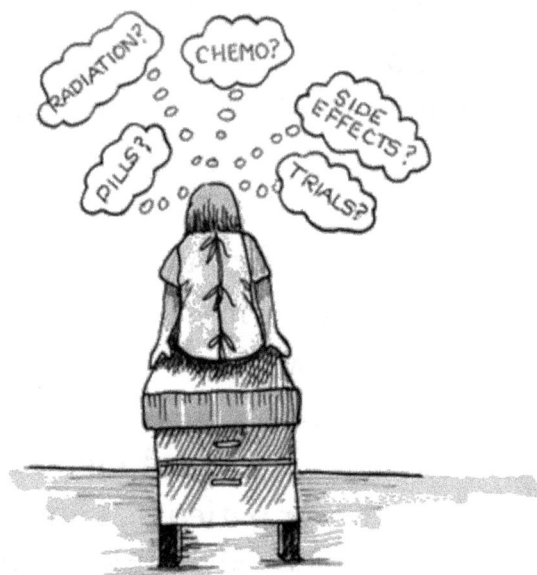

TRIALS AND CHOICES

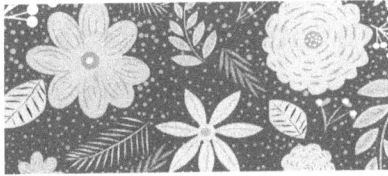

I was blessed with 8 great years
And then the cancer roared to life.
Was given many choices
To help with this new fight.

Learned about an exciting trial...
Combined a chemo with a pill.
Side effects were minimal
Which helped me conquer hills.

If it did not seem to work
Could quit at any time.
So took a chance it'd be the fit
Seemed worth it for my life.

Once again the medical staff
Were attentive and first rate.
They cheered me on and held their breath
That cancer would abate.

I was very fearful
To enter clinical trials.
But now my freedom's 7 years
I feel it was worthwhile.

This message is profusely clear
No two people are the same.
Our bodies are so different
Treatments can be changed.
Research all potentials and here's what I
would do
Choose treatments that you think will fit,
For # 1...
THAT'S YOU!

CHAPTER 6

~ FALL 2013 ~

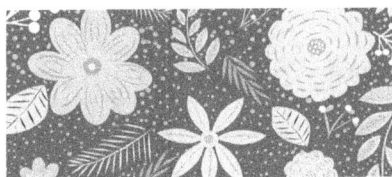

Uh Oh! Here we go again! The fact that I am adding a new chapter to my story is not good news. Three very important events took place in 2013. John retired in April, we took a family trip to Singapore to visit Dan and Sarah in July and my cancer recurred in September.

On Friday, September 13, I had a checkup at Mayo Clinic in Rochester, Minnesota. It had been an astonishing eight and a half years since my first ovarian cancer recurrence. According to statistics, once it returns, it usually comes back within half the time.

We held our breath and exhaled with each visit that the CA125 levels would stay low. But for some reason, I had a queasy feeling about this appointment and not because it was on Friday the 13th. I felt something was amiss in my abdominal area during the Minnesota Ovarian Cancer Alliance annual run the prior week. So, when the number rose from eight in March to 218, I was stunned and my shoulders shrunk into my body. I remember saying over and over again "I knew it". And the process began again.

First up was the all-telling Cat Scan. When the results came back showing a tumor in the liver, I was devastated. My doctor said that was actually a good thing because it could be cut-out and the liver would regenerate. Secondly, we had to find out when my very trusted surgeon and a liver specialist would be able to operate. We chose September 26 because John and I had our annual Vail vacation planned in between and our good friends Fay and Curt were to join us.

Secondly, we had an important choice to make concerning the drugs that would be used for therapy. My doctor was excited about a trial study that was available. It used a colon cancer chemo in tandem with an inhibitor pill that had promising synergy in combating ovarian cancer. If it did not seem to work, we could stop at any time and a traditional ovarian cancer chemotherapy would be used.

John and I agonized over the next two weeks, should we, or shouldn't we? Our decision had to be made by the time of surgery as an intra-peritoneal catheter would be inserted into my abdomen at the same time. Two days before surgery we took a chance and chose the trial study because that was the only way to get the combination of those exciting drugs.

After a wonderful week in Colorado we drove straight to LeeAnn's in Austin. It was September 25, the night before surgery and as we ate dinner at a Vietnamese restaurant I thought how strange and wonderful it was to be going through a normal routine at that time. I have to admit that it actually helped me from the typical "surgery fear factor".

In the early morning hours, we took off for Rochester. We were barely on the road when my cell phone rang about 6:00 a.m. It was my doctor telling me that I needed a chest x-ray and blood test prior to surgery to participate in the trial study. In a panicked voice I told her that there was not time as my surgery was scheduled for 10:00. She called back to tell me that it was pushed back to afternoon because of an emergency. It made John and me wonder if I should scrap the trial study. In the end, we decided to move forward, went through the requisite tests and were perched in a private room waiting for the nurse to bring me down to the operating room.

That was around noon and I was happy to get this new show on the road, have the surgery and recover enough to start the therapy. Every two hours a nurse would come into our room and tell us that the liver surgeon was not ready for me. My euphoria turned to fright and by around 7:00 p.m. I was in full blown panic mode. I could not stop crying and wondered how wide awake the surgeons could be at this late hour. It was not long until the surgeons were ready and John was allowed to accompany me to the next step. When my wonderful gynecologic surgeon entered the room to reassure me.

I remember saying, "You came to see me."

She smiled. "Of course I did," she said.

Surgery went well. The tumor was about two centimeters and was only leaning into the liver. Because it was cystic (very liquid) the chance of cancer cells escaping was high so my doctor washed out the abdominal area twice and turned over the organs to make sure there was no cancer lurking around.

Once again, I felt very fortunate to have the same, wonderful surgeon who treated John and me with dignity, respect and she even laughed at my crazy jokes! After giving her this story to peruse, she mentioned how much she enjoyed it and also learned a new word "dockling". I told her she can never retire.

One thing I learned about surgery after eight years is that things really do change, mostly for the better. Normally when I wake up from recovery there are so many drugs in my system that I am in one big stupor. So, how was it that when I opened my eyes John and Tim were sitting in front of me, plain as day?

Immediately, I thought something was

wrong as my body felt wonderful... no pain, haze or nausea. It was intoxicating to feel so good but scary, too!

My mind started racing as I began planning an early departure from those four walls. Knowing that I needed to walk to get out, and eat something to be able to walk, I asked the nurse what was available at this late hour. She said that anything could be ordered from the menu and would be delivered to my room. I was like a kid in a candy store and ordered graham crackers, chocolate milk and probably soup- had to eat something commensurate with just having surgery. After chowing down and feeling a little off kilter, I decided there is a reason you are started with Jell-O, broth, popsicles, etc. and then I mentally postponed my walk until morning.

The following day I was told that I had been given a three-day block in my abdomen, which explained the painless and stupor free wakening the night before.

Having Tim in my hospital room was reassuring, just like old times. With a smile, he handed me a beautiful decorated "Joy Jar" that Caitlin had made. She asked family and friends to send her fun memories of their time with me and she then typed them on colorful strips of paper. I decided to read one or two a day, but not surprisingly read them all at once. It was the perfect gift and I continue to read them from time to time, especially when feeling low.

The one person I could not bring myself to call about my new medical predicament was Jody as she was battling her own demons with her husband in the throes of early onset Alzheimer's. I wanted to find out what we were facing first and what our treatment plan would be, as she worries more than me.

When LeeAnn and her husband Jeff showed up the following day, she could not hide her delight at my appearance. Besides John, she has seen me at my absolute worst and thankfully keeps coming back for more. I turned to her for advice on how to tell Jody as I knew she would be devastated. LeeAnn assured me that she would understand and would be able to tell by my strong, coherent voice that I would be fine.

After walking the halls for two days, I was ready to leave. Unfortunately, nausea from the anesthesia was my biggest problem as the medical staff had a difficult time regulating it. Being alert and awake right away did have its drawbacks.

By the fourth day we were on our way home. Walking into a clean house with an abundance of food and gifts was truly unexpected. We had only told our closest friends and were surprised at the outpouring of good will. My birthday was the following week so Deb arranged a party at her townhouse. I received enough gifts in those two weeks to last a lifetime and soon learned that was just the beginning.

After a few weeks it was time to start the clinical trial. Each three-week cycle consisted of taking an inhibitor pill for ten days and receiving chemotherapy on days 3-5. Also, I had a cat scan every other cycle to see if the tumor was shrinking. The big catch to this study was that I had to physically be in Rochester, Minnesota for every cycle. It was not a problem while we stayed at our Minnesota home as we live only three hours away. It became a little burdensome while we were in Florida over six months.

Our friends thought it was crazy that we

could not receive the drugs at Mayo Clinic Jacksonville but we felt fortunate to be in the study and would follow the rules. In addition, my body tolerated the drugs and with the help of anti-nausea pills I was able to fly back and forth without any major problems.

There were to be six cycles but my blood count did not rebound quickly enough for the final chemo so that part ended after five. I relished the thought that the trial was over and my life would return to normal. For better or worse, my doctor approached the company distributing the inhibitor and the head of the study to see if I could continue with only the pills. The answer was yes, so we kept up the routine for the next year and a half. John became an expert at navigating air and car rental fares at a moment's notice as the pills still caused my blood levels to go down. We quickly learned that you cannot receive therapy if they are too low, regardless of the date of your airplane reservations!

During the two years I was in the clinical trial, my blood was tested every week. Although my old port worked sufficiently for the normal blood draw, it could not be used to inject dye during the cat scans. After several months of barely tolerating the digging for viable veins, I had enough and went under the knife to replace the old one. The super port allows dye to be injected... best decision I ever made! It does stick out more and is very noticeable but I have learned to put up with the stares from well-meaning people.

Things were going well when out of the blue, Mayo clinic implemented a structure change for the oncology department to become a team effort consisting of about five doctors, a nurse practitioner and others. I never knew which doctor would be seeing me until he/she walked through the door. It was disconcerting to me that if my cancer returned, I would be given the news from a doctor I barely knew. So, my caring oncologist allowed me to come in on days she was seeing patients. After a year on the study, this same doctor who had given me so much hope and comfort left Mayo Clinic to be closer to her Canadian family. John and I were heartbroken.

One December day, another doctor we had never seen before entered my examining room and I was not happy. But, while glancing at her notes she brought up the fact that we live in Florida over half the year and that all of her family members are huge Disney fans. My dismay immediately turned to excitement and she agreed to see me on the day she meets with oncology patients. We have great rapport and I have been seeing her ever since, always discussing the latest Disney changes for the first few minutes of my appointments.

Around that same time, John and I decided to stop the trial study for fear of the fallout from the seventeen cat scans I had in two years. The scans were used to measure tumor growth but fortunately for me, the tumor did not return so there was nothing to measure. My last cat scan was in December of 2015 and to my knowledge, the tumor has not returned. I was finally able to breathe a sigh of relief and happily accepted my new normal of once again being on the every "three-month" plan for doctor visits.

CHAPTER 7

~ 2018 ~

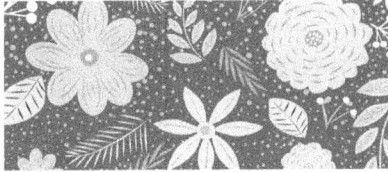

The greatest things I learned from my latest cancer experience are there are no boundaries for complete strangers to become very dear friends, old friends and family never forget you and the power of prayer is alive and well.

First of all, Jody, my sister who always insists on coming to help after each surgery no matter where we live or whatever time of year, arrived at Rochester the night before the first trial week ended. We had been staying at Hope Lodge, a wonderful facility for cancer patients who are being treated for any length of time, which is located across the street from the Mayo Clinic. It is enormous with multiple sleeping rooms, kitchens, dining rooms, living rooms and plenty of TVs ... just like being at home. We were truly grateful for the opportunity to stay and will never forget the kindness and hospitality from the staff.

Jody was able to sleep in our room that night and joined us at St. Mary's Hospital for my last blood draw of week one. Multiple nurses were involved in drawing the blood from my port on that day. They were about to give up when John noticed the blood was actually flowing through the tube.

After the nurses left with the blood sample, John announced that I had to get off the hospital bed so he could lie down. The other choice was to pick him up off the floor as he was in the process of fainting! Apparently, he could no longer watch me being worked on in any way, shape or form. We finally drove home, Jody stayed for the week and as usual, she spoiled me rotten ... just what I needed.

John and I had been living in Minnesota eight years when this latest health scare occurred. During that time, I met Fay who lived a mile away on our lake. What struck me was that she was taking in the beautiful sunshine in front of her cabin without a hair on her beautiful head. Walking past her, I quickly decided to go out of my "box".

"Are you a cancer survivor?" I asked.

She had a recurrence and was recuperating at her lake home. Suffice it to say that we bonded and she soon became a very special friend. I was thrilled when they built a permanent house on that site.

During my latest difficult stretch, Fay graced our home with enough homemade food to feed an army for a year, or longer. Every time we turned around there were homemade goodies, meals and an abundance of fresh vegetables from her garden sitting on our garage freezer or by our front door. My heart was overflowing from this angel that God brought into my life, just when I needed her the most.

I must also give a shout-out to all of our walking group members and neighbors from our Florida community. I am truly blessed with a multitude of new friends that somehow keep entering my life. Their concern for my precarious health situation is heartwarming and I feel immense gratitude for their fellowship during the winter months and for their emails and texts during the summers.

My "old" friends also took great care of me. Although Deb and Herb live in South Dakota they seemed to always be around with food and comfort. We spent our nights with LeeAnn and Kris in Austin before chemo and inhibitor treatments began, which provided a huge mental boost. We always left Kris and her husband Jeff's house with a grocery bag of, you guessed it, my favorite comfort foods; Teddy Grahams, caramel corn, boxes of cereal, hot tamales and more.

Of course, I would be remiss if my wonderful family was not mentioned. Their continuous support keeps me strong. Connecting with Dan and Tim each week is incredibly special. Watching them grow into caring adults with fulfilling lives of their own is what every parent dreams of. In fact, it was with immense gratitude that John and I were able to see our first grandchild, one-month old Miles, in Singapore for two weeks in April. Also, John and I celebrated our 40th wedding anniversary in May. Enough said about my soulmate.

I continue to be asked to talk to ovarian cancer patients. A friend recently gave me the phone number of her sister in law and asked if I would lend an ear and answer a few questions. After a three-hour conversation, we bonded through our shared experiences. I am not an expert and do not have a psychology degree but living with ovarian cancer seems to initiate one into a unique sisterhood with the ability to "get" what their members are going through. Feeling so alone in 2000 when I was first diagnosed, makes me feel compelled to help my "sisters". As I have said before, knowledge is power!

So, where does that leave me today, four and a half years since my latest recurrence?

My doctor visits are back to three months apart. I still get nervous before each one but that feeling prevents me from taking my health for granted and to truly appreciate every day. I am sincerely grateful to the medical community that works tirelessly for a cure for all cancers. The strides that have been made have given me hope that a cure can actually be a possibility.

For a survivor, hope is a wonderful thing!

SURVIVOR

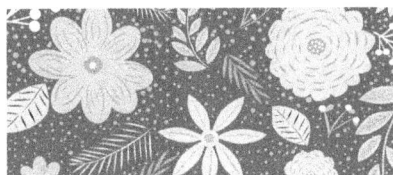

Cancer is a monster
Who takes your breath away.
Consumes with fear and woefulness
But does not have to stay.

Be mindful of all positive beliefs
To keep your essence safe.
Revere and cradle special thoughts
Creating a peaceful space.

Surround yourself with uplifting plans
Whatever brings a smile to you.
Remember that an all-out cry
Can benefit you, too.

Join some others with kindred needs
They'll likely give a call.
Ones you trust with honesty,
To carry over walls.

Last but not the least,
Look to family and your friends.
Focus on great memories
From past....to FUTURE ONES AHEAD!

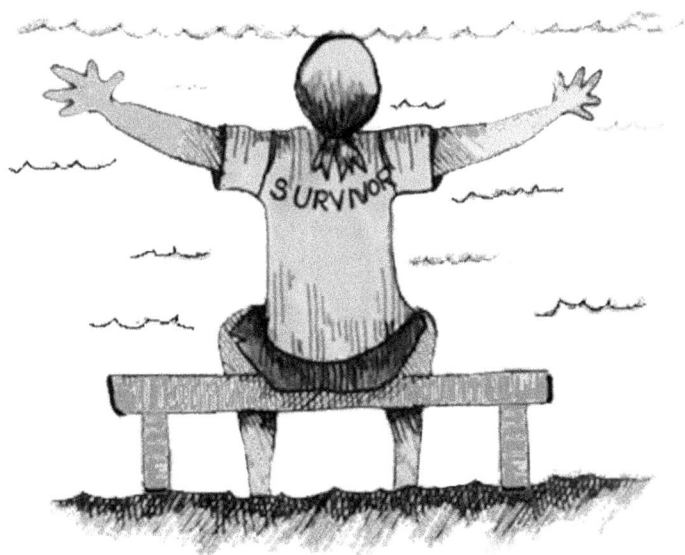

ABOUT THE AUTHOR

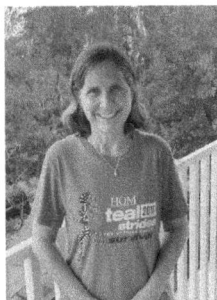

Jennifer Court was born and raised in Homewood, Illinois. She met her husband at a University of Illinois toga party in 1976 and they have been inseparable companions ever since.

While living in Wisconsin, Minnesota and Florida the last 43 years, the married couple expanded their family to include two incredible sons and daughter-in-laws. They are also the proud grandparents of three delightful grandsons.

Jennifer began writing *I Know What it's Like* around 2011 to enlighten her children about the details of her cancer "fight" that began in 2000. The story slowly morphed into a way to help other Ovarian Cancer survivors. In the process of being shared with others, Jennifer discovered that *I know What it's Like* has become a story of hope.

ACKNOWLEDGMENTS

To Sheila Tolbert who shared her beautiful artistic talents by illustrating several of my poems, throughout the story.

And to my wonderful family, friends and doctors who lifted me up, just when I needed them the most.

And thank you to Victoria Twead and Ant Press for publishing my book and helping me to get my story out for the whole world to read.

～

If you'd like to chat with the author and other memoir authors and readers, do join the friendly, fun Facebook group, We Love Memoirs.

https://www.facebook.com/
groups/welovememoirs/

ANT PRESS SURVIVAL STORIES

Do you have a survival story that would interest or inspire others? Would you like to see it published?

Write to Victoria Twead, at TopHen@ VictoriaTwead.com and she may be able to make your publishing dream come true.

Visit www.antpress.org to see more survival stories and publishing options.

www.ingramcontent.com/pod-product-compliance
Lightning Source LLC
Chambersburg PA
CBHW060250030426
42335CB00014B/1650